FALLEN

A Post-Concussion Memoir

Angela Lam

Gross Productions

Print ISBN: 979-8-991789530
E-Book ISBN: 979-8991789523

Author's Note

On New Year's Eve morning, I did the one thing experts always say is the worst thing that can happen to anyone over the age of fifty—I tripped and fell.

This is the story of what happened and how I learned to live with the repercussions of the fall while doing my best to get better. It is a fragmented story, told in bite-sized pieces, because that is how my mind works now. It is also fully illustrated with my original artwork, which is the primary way I've found healing and peace.

As is the nature of memoir, the book does not chronicle every incident that happened during my recovery and instead includes only those moments that serve to illustrate my story. This book is informed by journal entries, medical records, interviews with family and friends, and other information I've found while researching post-concussion syndrome and mild traumatic brain injury.

Some names have been changed or omitted to protect privacy. There are no composite characters. All dialogue is true to the personalities.

Brain Injury

How can we believe,
What we cannot see?
People wonder.
Think of the wind…
Invisible currents affecting
Depending on their strength
Clothes on a line swaying in a breeze
Leaves whispering and dancing
Hat blowing off
Weakened structures falling
Trees uprooting
We see the effects
But never the wind
Even wind chimes stir
When the invisible current flows
Like electrical impulses
In our tussled brain
Causing symptoms.

—Francene Gillis from Where Did i Go? a memoir plus

"Art makes the invisible visible."
¬*Paul Klee*

First Doctor's Appointment

I bring my list:

1. Pain in sinuses on left side where I fell on my nose and chin.
2. Ringing in the ears.
3. Nausea.
4. Disorientation.
5. Can't read. Can't focus on screens.
6. Extreme fatigue.
7. Can't walk more than 30 minutes without needing to rest.
8. Fitful sleep. Wake every 3 hours.

My primary care physician listens to the symptoms and nods. "You have a concussion," he says. "No reading and no screens for 10 days."

I gasp. "But I teach online, starting next week."

"You need to take time off work," he says. "I'll send a note home with you, okay?"

But it is not okay.

My husband listens while he slumps in the chair beside me. Last night, while lying in bed, I asked him to turn off the TV since the sound bothered me. "What's wrong? You can't tolerate TV anymore? What a pussy." Now he sits, chagrined, and I want to shake him and say, "See? I'm not a pussy. I have a concussion." But I don't say anything because my throat is closing, and my eyes are watering.

"When will she be back to normal?" my husband asks.

My primary care physician shrugs. "Anywhere from ten days to three months," he says. "That's the normal range for healing. We could do an MRI to see if there's anything else going on that would complicate a full recovery."

I want the MRI, but I don't ask for one. I don't know why. For some reason, I feel like everything I want to say or do is delayed for so long that by the time my body is ready to respond I can't remember what I was going to say or do anymore. And I don't know why. Why is my mind suddenly a blank chalkboard? Why is everything I think instantly erased?

"Come back in six weeks if you don't see any improvement, okay?" my primary care physician says. "We'll schedule an MRI at that time. Go home now and rest."

My husband and I leave with our arms dangling by our sides. Neither one of us reaches for the other. Neither one of us speaks. The walk to the car feels like forever with each step echoing in my ears.

Bardos

"You're always in the bardo," Pema Chödrön, a Buddhist nun, said during a talk. She told a story about a monk who went shopping before having lunch with a friend. "The shopping is a bardo," she said, "and having lunch with the friend was another bardo. You are not just in the bardo when you die. You are in the bardo now. You are always transitioning."

Every moment of life is a bardo.

My life before a concussion was a bardo. The concussion was a bardo. My life after the concussion was a bardo.

Where am I now?

Always in the bardo.

This writing is a bardo. Every word I yank from the depths of my mind is taking place in a bardo, the bardo of writing.

One way to stay in the moment, Pema said, is to remember you are always in a bardo.   .

As soon as you enter, you leave something behind. As soon as you leave, you enter something new. You are always entering and leaving, leaving and entering, moving from one moment to the next, always moving, moving, moving, breathing, breathing, breathing. Bardoing bardoing bardoing, if you take the noun and make it a verb.

Because of this constant state of momentum, you cannot afford to dwell in any experience beyond its lifecycle, for that would create stasis, an illusion of permanence the mind can cling to and create suffering.

All life does not have to be suffering.

We can liberate ourselves through living with the grace of a monk entering and leaving a bardo, shopping one moment, having lunch with a friend in the next moment, always focusing on the moment we are currently entering, not the moment we are leaving behind or the moment we will one day enter.

Just focus, right now, where you are, and you will experience freedom, freedom from the past over things you can't change and the worry about a future you can't control. You will plunge into the space of now, all of now and only now, and taste the beauty of it, all of it, before letting go and moving onward.

Turn this page, and the bardo of reading this story is over, and a new bardo of reading has begun.

Instant Karma

My daughter is the only one who knows what happened. Sure, there were bystanders—the PG&E technician inspecting a power line and a passing motorist who called out, "Are you all right?" as soon as my chin hit the asphalt and the headphones I was wearing flew off my head and landed thirty feet away along with the breakfast I was carrying. But the only person who knows what went on before, during, and after is my twenty-five-year-old daughter.

My daughter and I are sitting at the dining room table in the home I share with my husband. She is gazing intently at my face. I am telling her about the night before when I went to The Union Hotel with my husband to meet his guy friends, Mikey and Eric, for drinks.

Two hours and several drinks later, my husband slammed his napkin on the table and shouted, "Goddamn it!" The 49ers lost the last game of the year, and he wanted to leave immediately. He tossed what he had left in his wallet onto the table and shoved the bill at me. "Cover the rest, but don't put it on a card." He stormed out to use the restroom.

My body tensed as I opened my purse and rifled through the change I had. I had only been working part-time teaching novel writing, and the craft book I had written to supplement my income would not be released until next year. My eyes watered and my hands shook as I counted out what I had left.

"Is it enough?" I asked Mikey. My husband likes to leave a big tip.

Mikey shuffled the bills in his broad hands. "Don't worry. You've got it, sweetheart."

My husband returned before the server, and he tallied the money I had left. "Can't you do math? This isn't thirty percent." His face blanched white.

"Hey, hey, hey, big boy," Mikey said, moving his hands up and down. "Be happy with what you have—a beautiful wife who loves you."

My husband huffed and uncurled his fists. "You're right." He slapped Mikey on the back and motioned for me to follow him. "Let's go."

Mikey pulled me into a hug. "I love you, sweetheart."

"I love you, too," I said, squeezing him tight. Out of all my husband's friends, Mikey is the one I like the most. He cares about me like a little sister.

At home, my husband fell asleep, but I stayed awake, fuming. Anger radiated throughout my body like a furnace churning out heat. I didn't want to be stuck with the bill tomorrow night when we went to Graton Casino to celebrate New Year's Eve, so I planned to go for a run tomorrow morning and withdraw two hundred dollars in cash from the ATM.

The next morning was cold and frosty and dense with fog. I bundled up for a five-mile run. I didn't take my usual route to pick up the paper at my mother-in-law's house. I ran in the opposite direction, toward Montgomery Village, an outdoor mall between the high school and St. Eugene's Church. At the ATM, I shoved the cash into my zipped pocket and decided to take a shortcut to Whole Foods to grab breakfast too.

My phone rang through my headphones. It was my friend, Daniel, who lives in North Carolina, calling to catch up. I didn't want to talk to him while I was in the grocery store, so I let the call go to voicemail. Sometimes when I think about that morning, I wonder if I had just picked up the phone, talked to Daniel, and skipped the scones for breakfast, would I have avoided the accident? But I can't dwell on what could have, would have, should have happened. I can only tell my daughter what actually occurred.

"I was at the intersection of Hoen and Yulupa when the light turned green for me to cross, but as soon as I stepped off the curb, a car sped by, almost nicking me. I was so angry—from last night and the speeding motorist—that I started thinking I wanted everyone to die in a zombie apocalypse."

My daughter gasps. "Oh, no, those aren't good thoughts."

I nod, remembering. "At the next street crossing, I waited until the PG&E technician waved me ahead. I ran across, but tripped and fell on my jaw."

"Instant karma," my daughter says.

I tell her about the other times I've had bad thoughts during a run and how they always ended poorly, especially the time I was mulling over my frustration with being stuck caring for my dying girlfriend, Judy, while her husband went away for a golf tournament when I was stung in the head by a wasp. "Why don't I learn?"

My daughter rises and hugs me. "You need to forgive yourself and let go of those bad thoughts."

Closing my eyes, I breathe in her sweet scent. "I can't think anymore without my head hurting."

"That's the concussion," she says. "It'll get better."

I let her go. "I hope so," I say.

I Am Not What I Feel

Over the next several weeks, I cannot function. I do not sleep although I am tired. I do not exercise other than walking because it makes my symptoms worse—increased ringing in the ears, dizziness, and instability. My head feels like a fishbowl, full of water and ready to slosh over. I cannot eat solid foods because my teeth are loose. I spend my days watching the world go on around me or lying in bed with my eyes closed praying for sleep. Sometimes I drift off only to snap awake again, feeling worse than I did before I closed my eyes. The whole left side of my face is full of pain, from what feels like a knife stabbing my left eye to sinus congestion to a tightness in the jawline. Sometimes the back of my head hurts to the touch like it is swollen and tender.

All these symptoms put me on edge. I feel out of control. Without a filter, I spew whatever comes to mind out of my helpless mouth. I am combative, impulsive, rash. I spend time online shopping for things I do not want or need. I race out to the local market and buy expensive art I cannot afford. No one stops me. When the bills come, my hands shake and my chest pinches. How will I pay for these expenses without a job, without income? Will I ever go back to work?

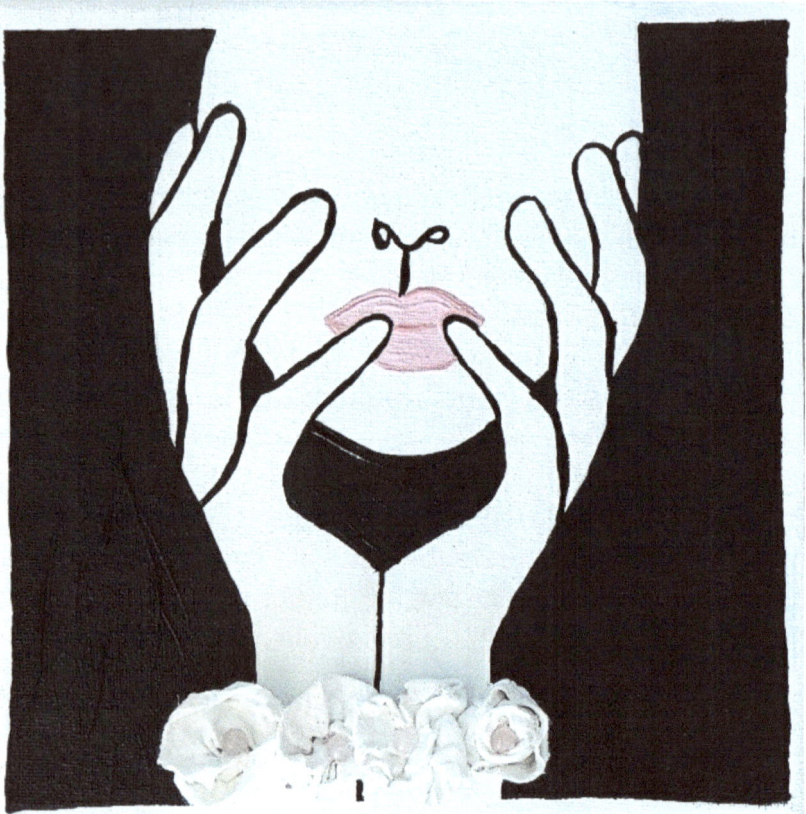

Diva #2, 8" X 8", mixed media

And the panic sparks another trigger-finger spending binge that only ends once I remove all my credit card information from my computer, my phone, and my wallet. I put everything in the safety deposit box at the bank. I ask the bank teller if I can make a special request to only access the security deposit box with my daughter present. The bank teller complies.

Now when I want to act out, I can't do what I had previously done. The items remain in the online shopping cart. The items are put back on shelves. I must sit with my feelings—

on the couch, in a store—and go beyond being out of control to examine the root of those impulses shooting from my damaged brain—anger, despondency, helpless, despair, self-pity, fear. Naming these feelings, one by one, I slowly untangle them from who I am, and the need to tamp down, extinguish, and kill those out-of-control emotions begins to wax and wane until I am not what I feel anymore. I am empty, hollow, broken, but no longer on a rampage to fill that empty, hollow, brokenness with things I do not want or do not need or cannot afford.

I just am.

Art Therapy 1

For Christmas, my daughter bought me two pocket-sized art journals. "For your purse," she said.

Smiling, I said, "Thank you." But I thought, *What a silly gift. Doesn't she know I don't paint on the go?*

Afterward, I tucked the two four-inch by four-inch books on a shelf behind my desk, never thinking of them again.

Then, in January, while I scrolled through Facebook searching for the online concussion support group my doctor recommended, I landed on an advertisement, "Journey with Color through Pocket-Sized Paintings." For twenty-five dollars, I could buy a self-paced course with a professional licensing artist and join an international community of fellow art students. With only fifteen minutes, the course promised I would complete a pocket- sized painting each day.

I signed up right away.

Every day for the next month, I religiously painted each assignment, from patterns to portraits in the style of Picasso to Matisse. Every painting was either built through layers or divided into segments and only took five minutes to complete. Within an hour, the paint would dry, and I could complete the next layer or segment. So, over the course of a day, in five-minute intervals, I finished one four-by-four-inch painting.

When the course was over, I enrolled in another one…and another…until I had purchased enough courses to fill one of the two pocket-sized art journals my daughter had gifted me on Christmas.

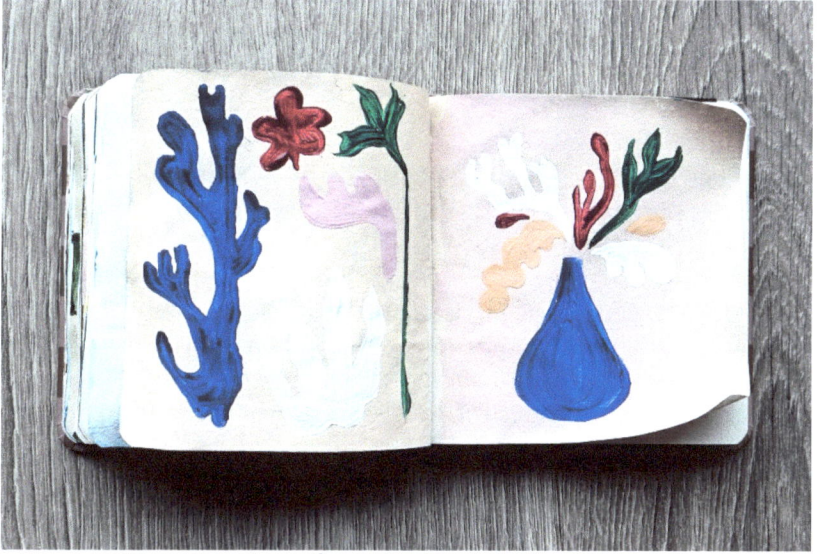

Two Paintings from My Pocket-Sized Journal

No Eating

When I couldn't close my jaw, I went to the dentist.

Not the emergency room, remembering a prior visit where I was told, "We don't do teeth."

Immediately after I jogged home after my fall, I sent a text message to the dental office explaining what had happened, and my dentist replied, "Come on in!"

When I arrived a couple of minutes later, I stumbled into the waiting room where I was waved back to an exam chair.

Dr. Kyle, going by his first name so as not to be identical to his father, whom he shared a practice with, leaned over my open mouth and probed with a metal instrument. "I think it's soft tissue damage," he said. "You'll probably be able to close your mouth in a few days."

"What about eating?"

"Only soup and smoothies," he said.

"Flossing?"

His eyes widened. "No, your teeth are loose. You don't want to yank them out."

I recalled another time when I had knocked one tooth loose after my jaw slipped while chewing a piece of steak on Valentine's Day. Now I had a whole mouthful of loose teeth, mostly on my lower jaw, but the panoramic x-ray of my mouth showed no fractured teeth or jawbone.

"You're lucky," Dr. Kyle said. "But you did go out with a bang for the new year!"

Beauty From Pain, Pain From Beauty

Over the next month, on a liquid diet, I lost over ten pounds. My husband said I looked good. I didn't want to tell him my trauma was his pleasure, but that's the way it sounded. Like women have dealt with the pain and humiliation of weight loss for men's pleasure over the centuries, from fad diets to not eating. I was barely eating, if you count the number of calories entering my body through butternut squash soup and banana protein shakes and hot tea to keep warm during January, the coldest month of the year. I longed for the day I could return to biting into anything solid without fear that my teeth wouldn't find purchase or worse that pain would sear through my jaw or the teeth would go sideways or whatever other dental horror might occur. I didn't think of my body, that shapely vessel of male desire, especially since it seemed like it wasn't such a priority after my husband's prostate cancer and my perimenopause. But it did matter. It does matter. It will always matter. Even when I am dead, if I am buried in a casket and not cremated or used as fertilizer for plants (yes, that's possible in Colorado), I will have to look good, meaning thin, young, beautiful. Who cares what I went through before dying. Beauty is paramount. It always is and always will be, won't it? It's enough to make me not want to be human, but a plant, with green leaves or a flower with delicate, perfumed petals, something ephemeral with the seasons, something not tied to a body. Something that does not have to worry about eating with a mouth and teeth and jaw that had been damaged from tripping and falling.

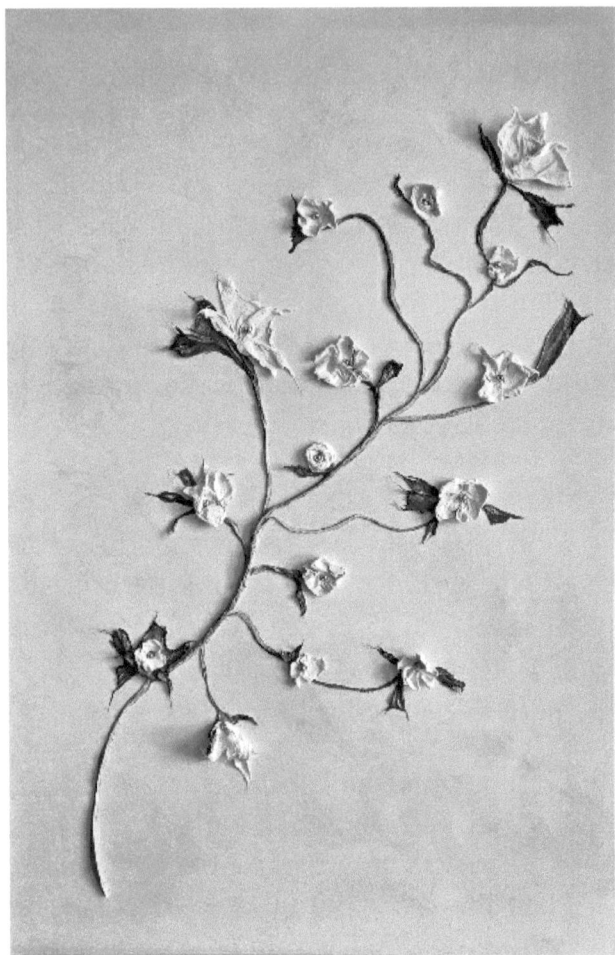

Blooming Branch, 36" X 24", mixed media

Loneliness

My father said, "You don't need friends. You have sisters."

True, but my sisters are scattered like dandelion dust across the United States:
    Utah,
        Texas,
            Virginia,
while I am stuck in Northern California, where I can't fly, the cabin pressure too tight against my skull, swelling my brain, leaving me reeling with dizziness and fatigue worse than vertigo, nor can I sail, the tossing and turning of the waves too much like the internal storm I weather each morning, stumbling back and forth on uneven feet, the keening weightlessness of a broken vestibular system.

I stay, a land mammal on solid ground, trying to connect with anyone in the outside world, so I don't feel alone, trapped between four walls, on the sofa, while my husband is away, but the phone calls and text messages I receive go unanswered, for the voices are too loud and the texts are too blurry, causing my stomach to pitch and my head to reel. So, I remain alone.

Double Vision

When I focus during yoga, I see double—two candles, two flames, two of everything. I blink, close my eyes, try again, but nothing changes.

My heartbeat ratchets in my chest, and my palms sweat. My head aches.

"What's the matter?" my husband asks.

I tell him, but he doesn't believe me. "How many fingers do I have?" he asks, holding up his hand.

The fingers waver and blur around the edges. I gulp. "Too many," I say. "I can't count that high."

He laughs, then stops. "You're serious."

Nodding, I feel tears fill my eyes. The whole world shimmers.

The doctor says it's part of the concussion. That when my body hit the pavement and my brain sloshed around in my skull, the intricate neural pathways short-circuited. "Rest," he says.

On the sofa, while closing my eyes, I wonder how long I will see things multiply and divide instead of coming together into one solid object, just as I feel shattered and scattered, a million pieces held together by this sack of ailing flesh, malfunctioning, useless, disassembled yet visually intact, as fragile as the light flickering against my lids.

Breathe

I'm not someone who enjoys long vacations or lazy days at the pool. I've been described as "aggressively ambitious." I want to write and publish a book a year and coach all my students to publication.

Lying on the sofa, with nothing to do, makes me feel sinful. I hear my father's voice in my head asking, "What you good for?"

"Nothing," I want to tell him, but he's been dead for seven years. I'm sure if I wanted to talk to him now, he would tell me to listen to the doctor. He spent the last decade or so of his life listening to doctors' advice to manage his Parkinson's disease.

My husband, who has been retired for just as long, says, "You can get used to doing nothing."

But right now, I only resent sitting on the sofa, closing my eyes, listening to Will on the meditation app I have installed on my phone telling me to focus on my breathing and nothing else. I am reminded of the days when I attended a silent retreat in New Mexico for one week, but I don't feel the same restless peace as I did then. I feel a wave of fear approaching, and my body tenses from my scalp to the soles of my feet. I try to relax, stop thinking, since it hurts to think, but I can only let go so far before the tide of unknowing tugs me back to shore.

Who will I become if I can't do anything I used to do, if all I can do is breathe?

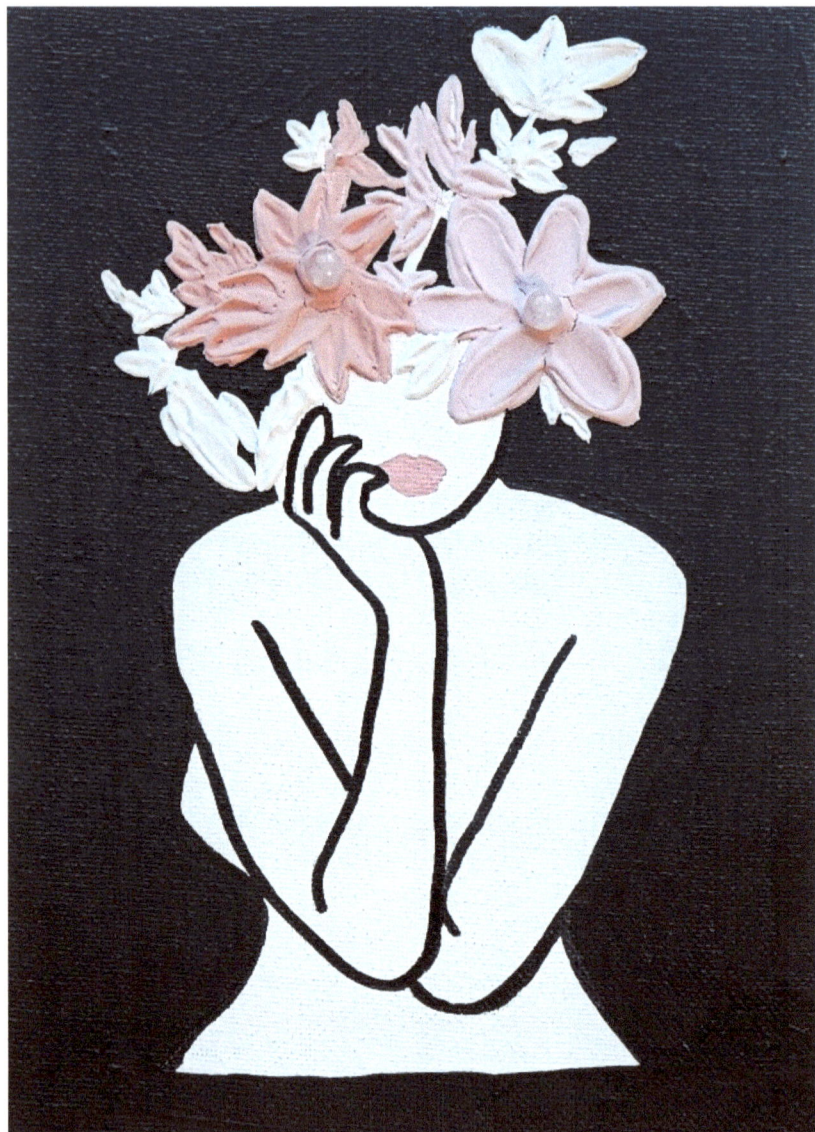

Diva #1, 8" X 8", mixed media

Read To Me

When the edits for a novel I started two years ago arrive, I panic. How will I stay on track for an October release if I can't read or write?

I call my ex-husband, the person I still turn to when life overwhelms me, and he offers a solution. "There's software I can install on your computer. It reads and writes for you. All you do is talk."

I exhale with relief.

Thankfully, I can talk.

The software is easy to use. As soon as I turn on my computer, I tell it what I want it to do, and it is done. I can sit in my office chair with my eyes closed and think of nothing. I can listen to the automated voice read the passage and I can accept or decline the editor's suggested changes.

Still, I can only work for fifteen minutes at a time, and those fifteen minutes cannot tally up to more than two hours a day or my head aches.

A month later, the edits are completed, and the novel is ready for pre-order.

A sense of relief and accomplishment strum through my body. For despite doctor's orders to do nothing, something has been done.

Headaches

The headaches do not start until after the MRI results. I have micro bleeding in the right parietal lobe of my brain.

All day searing pain radiates from the back of my skull. I can only take Extra Strength Tylenol since Motrin might have caused the bleeding in the brain, some side effect from ibuprofen that the dentist did not know and the doctor did not tell me.

Years ago, my best friend suffered from a buildup of fluid in the brain. He had to have surgery to restore equilibrium. After the surgery, he lived with a shunt in the back of his skull until the fluid completely drained. For over a year, he lived, unemployed, with his mother.

I cannot sleep. I am worried I will be like him, unwillingly dependent for over a year.

When the pain will not leave, and my head continues to feel full, I go to the beauty salon and ask the beautician to cut off my hair. Half an hour later, I am five pounds lighter. I no longer feel like I am balancing an aquarium on my neck.

But the throbbing headaches only weaken. They do not go away, not until much later, after asking for good thoughts and kind prayers from family and friends.

By my next doctor's appointment six weeks later, the headaches have subsided along with the internal bleeding.

I do not need surgery.

Relieved, I thank everyone for their prayers and thank God

for listening to them.

Here is a picture from that time—cropped hair, stylish and manly, an urbane commentary hiding a secret history only those close to me know, while the rest of the world just sees a middle-aged woman embracing her age through the statement of short hair.

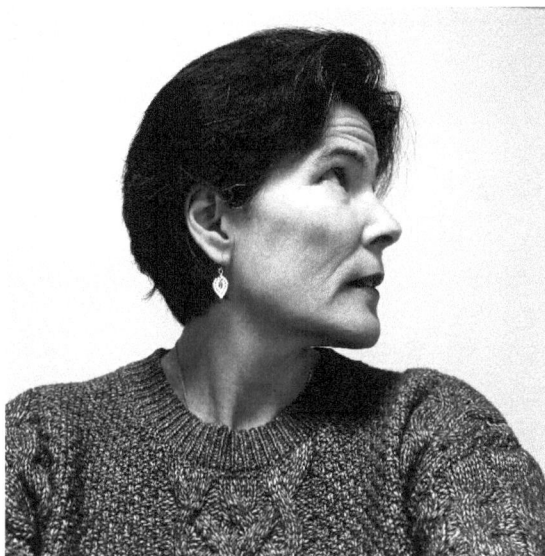

Self-portrait

The Body Does Not Speak English

Or French, or Spanish, or Swahili.
The body speaks through physical sensations:
Heat and cold, soft and hard, smooth and prickly.
Breathing opens the channel of communication.
Art translates what the body feels into something
The world can see and understand.

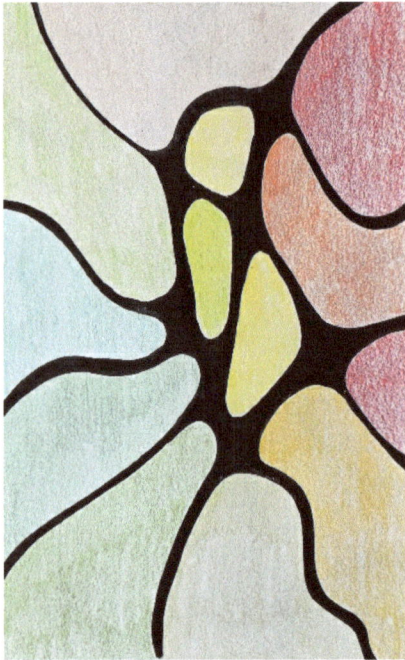

Nebulous, 8" X 10", Neurographic Art

Art calms the nervous system, relaxes the body,
Promotes healing. Art rewires the brain through
Neuroplasticity. How? The act of making art creates
Neural connections in the brain, bridging what has died
With something new and alive.

Art reduces stress, promotes mindfulness,
increases awareness, regulates emotion,
processes trauma, and improves mental health.

The brain and creativity interact to promote healing.

The Art Of Doing Nothing

I used to be a morning person. I would wake before dawn, run for one hour, watch the sunrise, stretch, eat breakfast, and take a long, hot bath before working.

My husband used to say I accomplished more in the first three hours of waking than he did all day.

Now all of that is untrue.

I am not a morning person. I wake up, head swimming, eyes stabbing with pain, feet heavy with no balance. I turn over, but I can't fall back to sleep. I can't sleep more than an hour at a time, and those hours don't add up to enough.

When I finally rise, I sit on the sofa and listen to a meditation app for one hour. I do nothing but listen and breathe.

No need to empty my mind or wrestle with thoughts.

My mind is already empty.

I no longer think.
I am a body on a sofa with no mind.

I am a hollowed-out shell.

I am nothingness.

As soon as the hour is up, I stand and stretch and make a cup of coffee. I sit on the stoop outside the front door and watch the sun rise. I go back inside and make breakfast which is a protein shake since I cannot chew. My teeth are still loose.

The old me would be writing. The new me goes into the

family room and stares at a canvas. She considers the shape of her feelings, sculpts something three dimensional on the flat surface. She lets her hands get sticky and dirty and hard with joint compound as she kneads the fabric. Fifteen minutes go by, and the timer on the oven bleeps. Hands washed and dried, she sets the timer for another fifteen minutes, and she goes outside for a walk around the block. She traces the path she once used as a warm-up for her morning runs, but she feels her chest pinch and her eyes water. Her lungs remain flat against the air where they once inflated like tires or balloons.

The world hasn't changed, but she has.

When she returns home, she resets the timer for fifteen minutes. She returns to the canvas to see how much she can sculpt before the fabric hardens. After one hour of art, she must stop for the day. Her eyes are throbbing, and her arms are heavy with fatigue. She lies down, closes her eyes, listens to another meditation app, and tries to nap for an hour. The rest of the day she does nothing, and that nothingness starts to define her in ways she never imagined. She becomes nothing, and nothing is her.

Fair-Weather Friend

Finally, someone arrives. The blue minivan pulls up to the curb. A stout woman wearing stylish clothes descends from the driver's side.

"Emma's here!" I call over my shoulder to my husband who is working at the back of the house, preparing it for sale.

I met Emma during an author event at Copperfield's bookstore over a year ago. We usually get together once a month to share a meal and our writing.

We haven't seen each other since the holidays.

After a brisk hug in my warm kitchen, Emma hustles me outside.

My husband bustles out the front door, exclaiming, "But we haven't met!"

Over the purr of the engine, Emma extends her arm across my body to grasp my husband's hand poking through the open window. "I'll have her back in a few hours," she promises.

As soon as we pull away from the curb, I remind her I can't stay out for over an hour, or my body becomes tense, my eyes blur, my ears ring, and fatigue pools around my limbs until I am curled into a ball.

"Okay, one hour," she says, although the look on her face doesn't confirm she understands this information.

We drive to our usual haunt, a chain restaurant that serves breakfast all day, and sit at our usual table, with me on the bench and Emma on the chair, the abstract paintings I love hung above us like perpetual evening stars. I order a bowl of tomato soup and a cup of tea, no cream or sugar.

"That's it?" she asks. "Why, you'll starve to death."

I remind her I haven't been eating solid food for months, and my weight loss has plateaued. I can still fit into my clothes, although I no longer fit into my life.

Emma is talkative, as usual, but today her voice sounds like a beehive buzzing between my ears. All around us, in the mostly empty restaurant, a magnitude of chatter rises, from the clatter of utensils, the rattle of bussed tables, to the hum of conversations. I breathe deeply, try to focus.

Emma removes a sheaf of paper from her purse. "Can you edit these?" she asks, sliding them along with a red pen across the table.

The words swim like black worms in white milk, and my stomach pitches. "No, I can't," I say. "My vision is still blurred."

"But it's been months," Emma says.

I shrug. "The doctor said it could take up to two years for me to return to my baseline."

She nibbles on her lower lip, and her gaze darts anxiously from side-to-side. "Aren't you working?"

Although I am not teaching a class, I have two students I am mentoring. "My ex-husband installed software on my computer that reads to me. I can talk to it, and tell it what to type. That's how I've managed working."

"Oh," she says with a crestfallen expression. She snatches

back the pages. "I'll read to you, and you can tell me what to change."

"Not here," I say, waving a hand around the air above my head. "It's too noisy."

"We can go outside," she suggests.

But the air is too cold, and the heaters aren't working.

Back at our table, the server delivers our meals.

Emma tucks her pages back into her purse. "Oh, well, next time." Her sigh is pregnant with disappointment. She picks up her fork, forces a smile. "So, tell me what's new."

Between sips of soup, I share the litany of complaints from my body, the endless resistance I receive from the health insurance company, and the list of specialists I'm still waiting to see.

She scrunches her nose and changes the subject to something more benign—her daughters. The eldest is living with her boyfriend and filming a documentary. The youngest is an artist working for a local grocery store while moonlighting as a costume designer for a nonprofit theater. The lighthearted stories fizz in my head like champagne bubbles. I get drunk on her daughters' lives—young, healthy, full of potential—that I forget to finish my soup. Even my tea gets cold.

But my body can't keep up with the information. The stories jumble and bunch up, twist into knots. The facts don't line up anymore, and I glance at my watch. "I have to go soon," I say. "I need to take a nap."

"Oh, okay," she says, staring at her half-eaten plate. Usually,

Emma takes three hours to finish a meal.

After the leftovers are boxed and the bill and tip are paid, we leave.

Outside, the sunshine screams into my eyes. I slide the amber-tinted glasses up the bridge of my nose and slide into the passenger seat of the minivan. Emma chatters some more, but her voice drips and dribbles as we near my home. There is so much to say, and not enough time. But my head is full, and my body is achy. I feel depleted, exhausted, worn out like I just climbed a mountain instead of sitting in a restaurant sharing a meal with a friend.

By the time I close the front door, and Emma has zipped away, a mix of relief and hollowness fills the room.

A part of me doubts I will see her again.

The immediate sigh of her absence is slowly replaced by a more pressing matter—the gaping hole she will leave in my life.

I know people will say, "No friend is better than a bad friend," and those people will text or call with their condolences instead of stopping by for a visit.

As I stand in the living room, I feel empty. I want to fill that emptiness with anyone or anything, so I don't have to confront the vacancy in my life or the fact that I am useless.

State Of Mind

A long time ago in a faraway place I lived with my husband and his dog, Sophie. When Sophie was dying, I enrolled us in a spiritual class with the Buddhist nun, Pema Chödrön, called, "This Sacred Journey." I wanted to learn how to move through the bardo of living through the bardo of dying to help Sophie transition to the next life. One of the sacred reminders I printed out and posted next to my computer read, "You are going to die, and all you'll take with you is your state of mind."

For a long time, I believed this sacred truth. I believed in the permanence of the mind in a world where everything would eventually fall away. But when I hit my jaw on the pavement and lost my mind, I realized this maxim wasn't true for my experience. The mind, like the body, would die. Whatever remained was not the body or the mind. It was something else. Something for which I have no words.

Consciousness no longer held the same weight as it once did. When I tried to connect with my intuition, I encountered nothing but static. Occasionally, if I concentrated, I could catch a moment of clarity like hearing a voice on the radio while tuning into and out of a frequency. But most of the time, I could not make sense of anything. The sixth eye, located between my two physical eyes, had been damaged just as badly as my ordinary vision. Everything in my body, from my head to my feet and all the parts in between, had short-circuited after my brain sloshed inside my skull like a bowl of Jell-O.

It took months before the static cleared, and I could reconnect with my intuition. For the longest time, I feared it would never happen. During those days, I felt disconnected from God, which reminded me of a story I had heard about hell being the absence of God, not the presence of the devil. I felt the absence of God during the worst moments of my recovery.

So, I took down that sacred reminder and cut around the words, "state of mind," and placed it in a piece of art I created to express what it felt like to have a concussion. I tore out hands in Michaelangelo's painting, *The Creation of Adam*, and placed them above and below a profile of a head with a shadow profile facing the opposite direction to express confusion. I fixed gold leaf in lightning bolts across the background to illuminate that moment of impact, both at the back of the head where the damage occurred and diagonally across the head to show the ripple effect throughout the entire mind.

While other people in my post-concussion support group expressed connecting more deeply with God after a mild traumatic brain injury, which is what a concussion is, my experience has been different. I felt that tenuous energetic thread fray between God and myself, and the threat of losing all connection with my Higher Power scared me.

Thankfully, that connection, that frequency, that divine integration has been restored.

But I will forever question whether the only thing we take with us when we die is our state of mind.

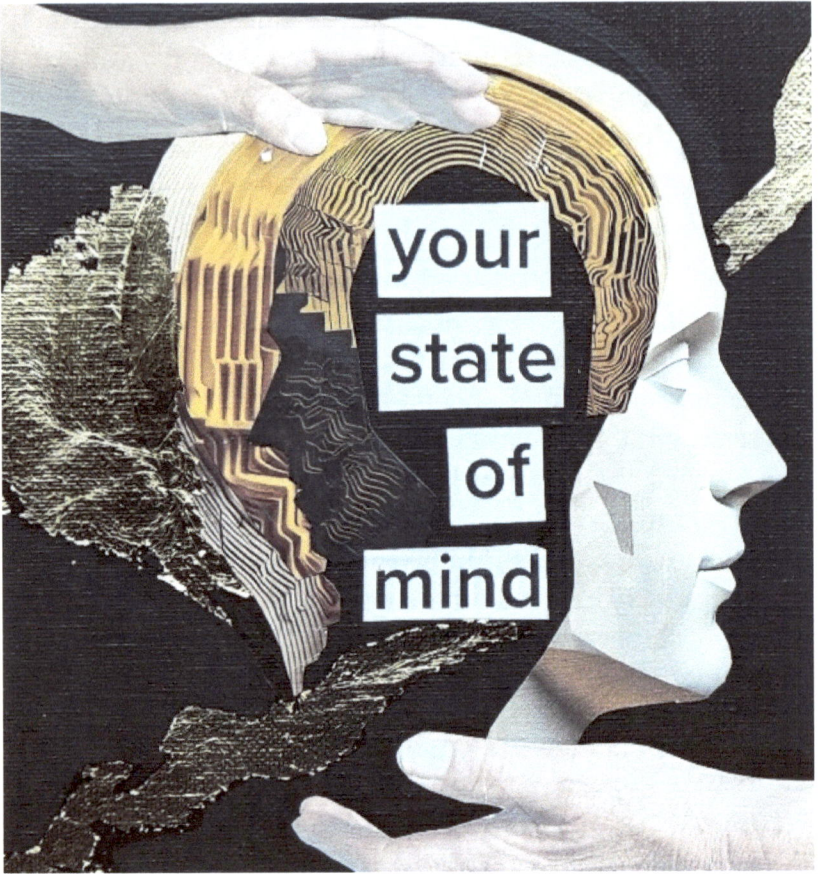

State of Mind, 8" X 8", mixed media

Walking

Twice a day, I go for walks with my husband. We stroll through the neighborhood for a half hour each time, holding hands, observing nature. From the tiny buds of the lantana plants (purple, yellow, red, and white) to the flowering bougainvillea in our yard, we ooh and ahh over the world waking up. We walk through all seasons—from the bitterness of winter (scarves and gloves and hats, oh my) to the mildness of spring (long sleeved T-shirts and jeans) to the afterglow of summer (strolling in tank tops and shorts after the sun has set) to the bite of autumn with its blustery days and hint of death (layers, layers, layers). We amble through parks, over bridges, beside creeks, and through shopping centers in old neighborhoods and new subdivisions. Our love for each other soothes one another after the monotony of illness, the comfort of routine, and the constancy of changing weather. Our walks are the highlight of my days, the bright spot of my eternal future, and the one thing that I can count on to make me feel better no matter what condition I wake (dizzy and full-headed or clear-eyed and focused). These forays into the natural world remind me I am one with nature. I am part of the cycle of life, the river of healing, the order of the universe.

Bionic Hearing

I lie awake at night listening to the sounds no one else hears: scurry of rat feet, zap of electricity from the mouse trap, snap of a twig from the neighbor's yard. Of course, I can't sleep with the cacophony of life going on around me. But my husband slumbers, unaware, of the activity surrounding us.

In the daytime, normal sounds bother me. I cringe when I answer the phone. Everyone's voice is a singer at a rock concert screaming over wailing guitars. My husband's cooking sounds like an out-of-tune orchestra: clink of silverware against edge of pot, clang of oven door, beep of timer. Dinner is done.

It is never silent. Even when sound leaves around me, it rises within me. My ears buzz with an annoying hum like TV static, like nails on chalkboards, like a tinny bell rung repeatedly. It is the only sound I can't escape, the only sound that echoes my sickness, the only sound I wonder and fear I'll have to endure forever.

Role Reversal

I drive my daughter to the Thai restaurant
To celebrate her twenty-fifth birthday.

She grips the "oh-shit" handle above the door,
Says, "Pull over. I'll drive."

I slide to a stop too close to the curb
On my residential street.

Shame pours over me like sweat,
And I shake like a soundless rattle.

"You're okay," my daughter says.
"You just don't need to drive right now."

She steps outside, circles the car,
Waits for me to get out.

I remember eight years ago
Telling her the same thing

As she ran my white Saturn up the curb,
Almost knocking over the cypress tree.

Now she steers smoothly, brakes evenly,
Parks perfectly outside the restaurant.

She even has the correct change for the parking meter.
Beside her, I feel like a child with a big purse.

Inside, we take the elevator, no stairs.
"I don't want you tripping again," she whispers.

The restaurant is quiet. We are the only patrons.
While waiting for our meals, we pose

In front of the koi pond and take selfies.
The owners say we look alike—same slanted eyes.

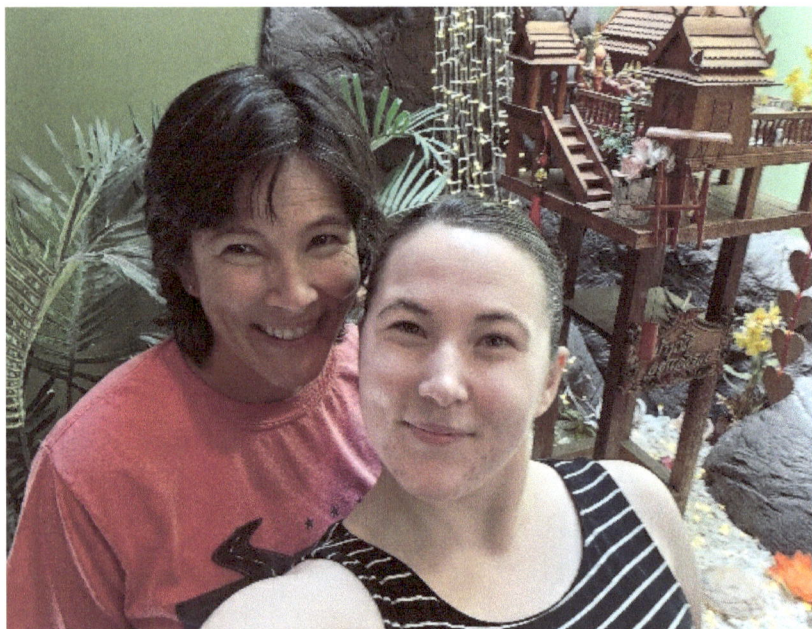

My daughter, Rose (right), and me (left)

But we are so different. She tells me about work,
About married life, about her dogs.

I tell her about waiting for an appointment
For a neuro-ophthalmologist, my self-appointed art therapy.

I scroll through and show her everything I've done:
Dolls with sculpted dresses, flowers molded out of clay.

She nods and listens, ever patient,
Like her father whom I miss at times like this.

I move my noodles around my plate with my chopsticks,

Ask for a takeout box for leftovers, and pay the bill.

Outside the winter sky burnishes like a metal bowl,
And tiny crocuses dot the meridian—spring is near.

"I love you, Mama," my daughter says,
hugging me outside my home.

"I love you, too, Chickey," I say, squeezing her close, smelling her apple-scented shampoo.

Tears prick my eyes, and my nose feels full.
But I don't cry as she drives away.

The Faults Of The Child Revisited Upon The Adult

The neurological ophthalmologist insists on examining the MRI. "I want to see the empirical data," he says, as if he knows better than a trained technician.

After a trip to the radiologist and a release form signed, I am given a CD-copy which I deliver to the eye clinic. I am told to go home and wait. The doctor will call me in one hour.

He does. "From what I can see, the injury looks too old to be from this fall. Have you ever fallen when you were younger?"

I think back and remember. Elementary school. I must have been eight, nine or ten. Mom was working at the bank. My sisters were inside watching cartoons. In the backyard, I climbed to the top of the swing set. I performed a trick I learned at school, swinging around, then letting go, thinking I would land on my feet. But I didn't. I fell on the back of my head on the concrete, not the grass. I stared up at the sky, blinked a few times, then scrambled to my feet. I wondered, *What went wrong?* I didn't know the physics behind why a stunt you could do from a bar three feet off the tanbark could not be duplicated from a bar seven feet off the ground. All I knew was the sting of failure.

I rubbed the back of my head. *Was I okay?* I walked into the house and wandered around my bedroom. I don't remember a headache or dizziness or nausea. Nothing out of the ordinary. I didn't even tell my mother about the fall after she came home from work. I acted as if nothing had happened.

Forty plus years later, I am recalling that disastrous trick on the top of the swing set and how I hit the back of my head on the concrete. If that is the accident that caused the micro bleeding, then why didn't I have any symptoms like I do now?

I realize the doctor is waiting for a response. But all I feel is the hot shame of failing. If I admit my fault as a child, will it negate the help that I need now? I steel my back and repeat what my primary care physician told me—the micro bleeding was from this fall.

The doctor sighs. "Then I will refer you to rehab," he says.

Tears of relief spring to my eyes. That fallen child, never seen, has allowed the injured adult to finally receive the help needed to get better.

Talk Therapy 1

Over the video conferencing software, Peter stares at me with his owl-like eyes and rocks back and forth like he's sitting in an invisible rocking chair. He tells me about his decision to sell his house and purchase a recreation vehicle and drive up to Alaska where he is camping until the end of summer with his rescue dog, Finnegan.

I don't tell him I have a character named Finnegan in one of my books about superheroes, which is strange because since the concussion, my mind has no filter. Thoughts shoot out like fireworks—bang, bang, bang—and the sky between me and everyone else lights up with things I should not say, things people don't want to hear.

Except now. Now I'm listening.

"Healing is a river," Peter says. "You can't move a river."

I sit before the computer monitor watching and listening even though I've been advised to avoid screens. But I can't find a psychologist who takes patients in person that my insurance will cover, so I am stuck here, with Peter, for fifty-five minutes once every two weeks.

"Even if you can't feel or see any improvement, underneath it all, you are healing," Peter says. "Trust the process."

In between our appointments, I try to trust the invisible healing river coursing through my brain. I continue to meditate, pray, walk, and rest, even as I struggle day-to-day with securing other appointments—physical therapy, occupational therapy, speech therapy, vision therapy, and vestibular therapy—so I can once again be whole.

Schurig Center

My writing buddy, Nicole, stops by the house to visit. She sits on the green sofa and talks about her nephew who recovered from a concussion with help from the Schurig Center.

I call the number and leave a message. Days pass. No response.

"Try their website," Nicole suggests.

Oh, the irony. The medical community advocates avoiding screens to promote healing. But to access professional help you need a computer.

I leave an email requesting a phone call.

A week later, while I am driving to pick up the newspaper at my mother-in-law's house, my phone rings. I pull over and turn off the engine and speak for fifteen exhausting minutes with a volunteer who explains the services offered. Out of everything available, I am only interested in concussion care. "I'll put you on the waiting list," the volunteer says. "The group meets once a week for three hours online."

Three hours? Online? I can't do anything for three hours. My eyes tire after fifteen minutes while working online. There is no way I can participate in the program.

"If you're interested, you can come to our facility in Marin and take art therapy once a week," the volunteer says. "I could have an in-take coordinator meet with you."

"How long would that take?" I ask.

"One hour online."

Oh, no. Not online again.

But I am polite. I ask, "And how long are the art therapy sessions?"

"Thirty minutes."

The drive to Marin is one hour. My husband would have to drive, since I am uncomfortable going any farther than five miles from our house. He would have to wait thirty minutes while I participated in art therapy, then he would have to drive another hour to get home. I think about my fifteen-minute pocket-sized paintings. "No thanks. I'm already doing art therapy at home."

When Nicole asks about my experience with the Schurig Center, I tell her everything. "That's too bad," she says. "But I'm glad you're getting help from something."

That something is art. I don't know the science behind it (though I've been told it calms the nervous system and rewires neural pathways), but I do know how I feel when I paint—free from limitations and completely at peace.

Art Therapy 2

My obsession with Barbie started as a young girl.

In between watching cartoons with my younger sisters, Cynthia and Elizabeth, the commercials grabbed my attention with the catchy tune, "We girls can do anything, right Barbie?"

And my sisters and I would respond, "Right, Barbie!"

In the commercial, Barbie swaggered on stage dressed in a business suit and briefcase, then disappeared for a few moments before she reemerged in an evening gown. Work, first, then the opera. I wanted to be Barbie—fiercely independent and incredibly glamorous and desired by the hottest guy in town, Ken.

During my concussion recovery, I flipped through photographs I had taken during a previous visit with my sister, Cynthia, in Texas. At an indoor flea market, I traveled from stall-to-stall photographing original artwork that I admired but could not afford. When I spied a three-dimensional bust on canvas, I cried, "I want to do that!" But as soon as I returned from the trip, I placed that thought on the backburner of someday.

Someday was now.

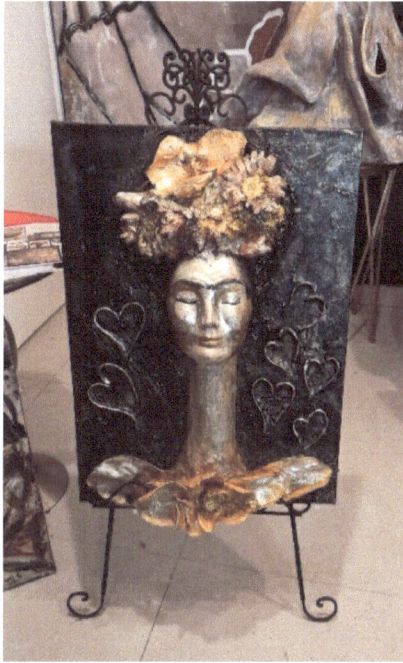

Mixed Media Artwork by Yesenia Garza

Cynthia offered to send life-sized torsos from her hairstyling class, but I settled on premade cake pics. I preferred working with the closest thing I could get to an actual Barbie—doll-sized plastic sculpted torsos, arms, face, and artificial hair, minus the posable legs.

Working fifteen-minute intervals, up to one hour a day, I fastened the back of each cake pic to a canvas using fluid matte medium. With a wad of brown butcher's paper, I sculpted the resemblance of a skirt. Later, I draped cloth dipped in joint compound over it. I pinched folds and ruffles into the skirt, smoothed the material over waist and breasts. I left the arms bare.

I waited two days for the dress to harden before I painted

and varnished the entire artwork with gloss gel medium.

I made the first doll art for me and titled the work, *Arianna at the Ball.*

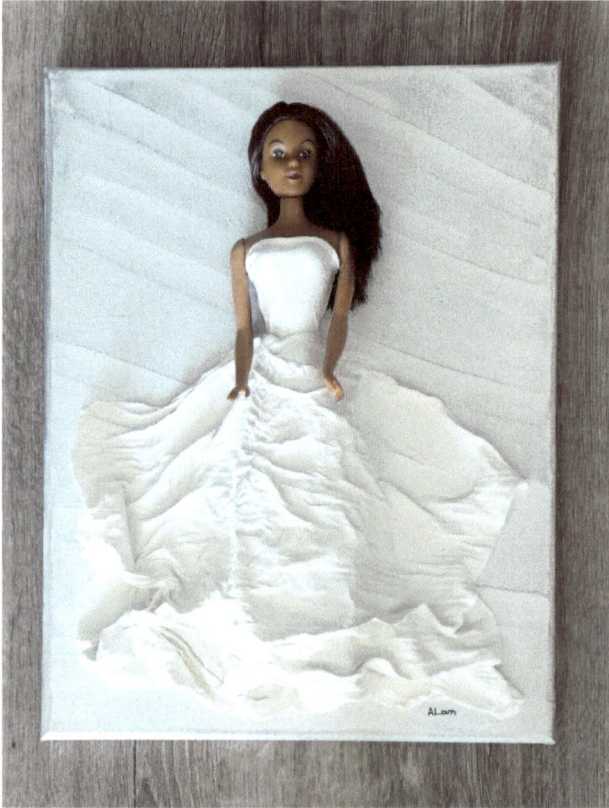

Arianna at the Ball, 14" X 11", mixed media

Arianna's cake pic came with a twin who I named Destiny. She had a haughty tilt to her mouth and a shinier gloss to her hair. I knew she would want something more dramatic, so I sketched out something sleek and modern. After much consideration, I settled on a blue, body-hugging evening gown against a silver and sapphire background.

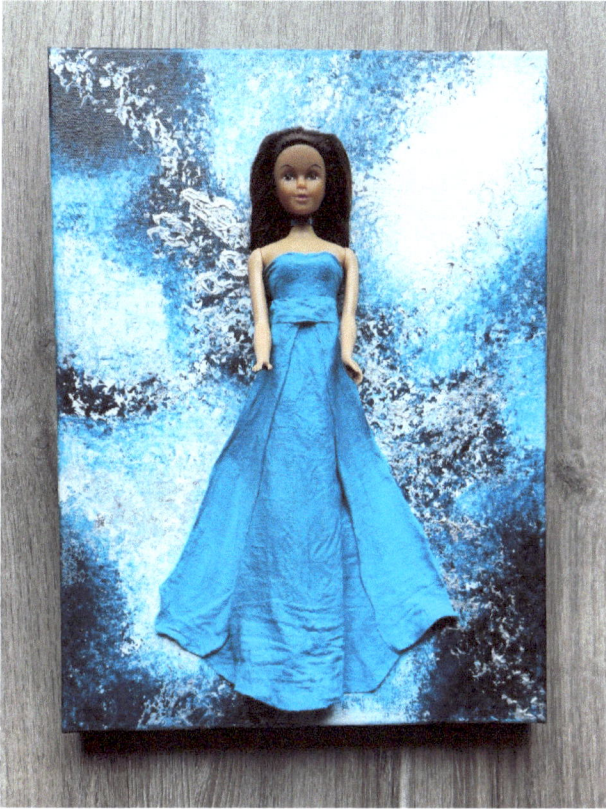

Destiny, 14" X 11", mixed media

Next, I fashioned a buxom blonde in yellow for Cynthia, and shipped the doll art to Texas.

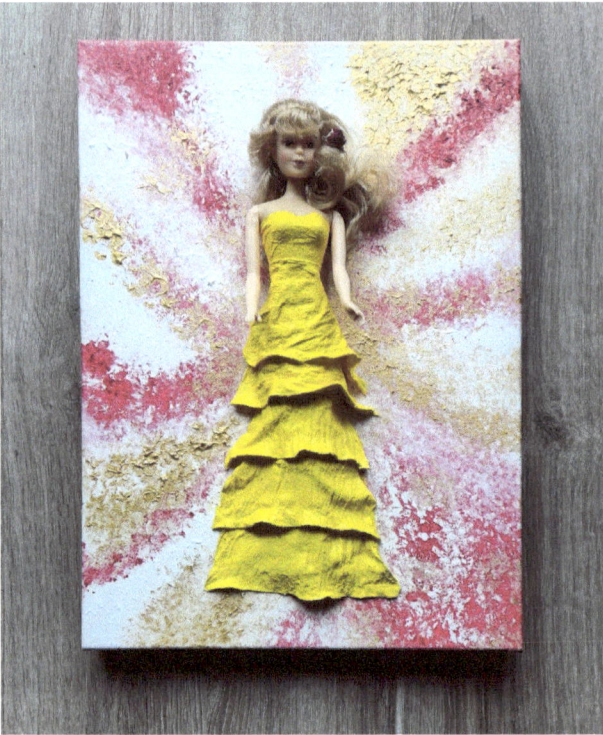

Cynthia's Doll, 14" X 11", mixed media

Finally, I spent several weeks making an image of the Immaculate Heart of Mary for my sister, Elizabeth, a consecrated virgin who cares for my elderly mother. She was also the sister who sent the Immaculate Heart of Mary medal to me, blessed by the Pope. She promised to pray for the bleeding in my brain to heal without surgery. When I saw the doctor twelve weeks after the accident, he told me the bleeding had stopped. God may have answered our prayers, but Elizabeth was the one who prayed the hardest. I wanted this doll to be extra special for her.

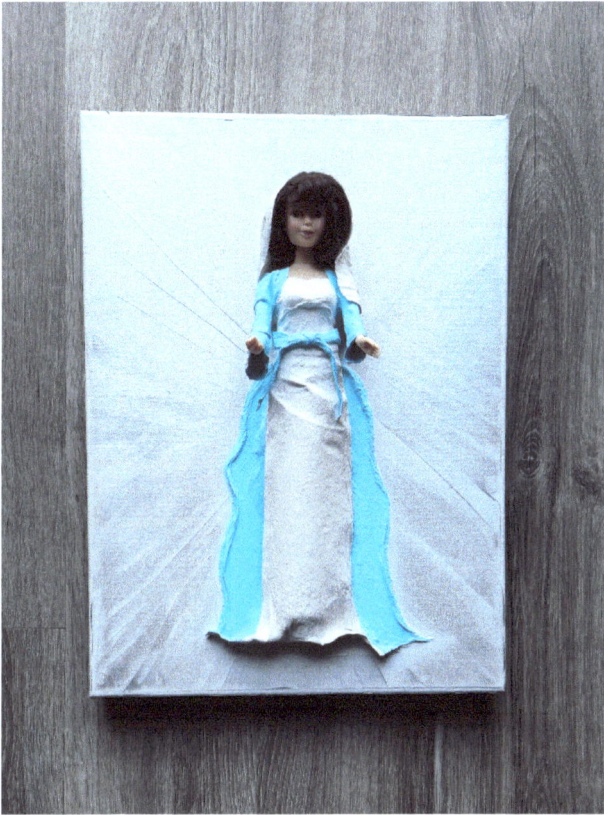

Immaculate Heart of Mary, 14" X 11", mixed media

Finally, I shipped the doll art to my sister's home and anxiously awaited her response.

Shortly after receiving confirmation from the carrier that the package had been delivered, I received an email from Elizabeth:

"Thank you very much for sharing your time and talent with me. We have so much to be thankful for as God is the one who answered our prayers through the intersession of his Mother."

While my doll art is nothing compared with Yesenia Garza's stunning style, it is an expression of my love for Barbie and my sisters.

Neurological Rehabilitation

"I'm sorry, but your referral was declined," a sour-sounding woman says over the phone.

"What do you mean by declined?" I ask. "How can my insurance company decline a medically approved service?"

"The referral is coded all wrong," the woman says.

Tears fill my eyes. An administrative error is preventing me from receiving the services I need to get well. "What can I do?"

The woman rattles off a list of numbers and letters and medical terminology that sounds like nonsensical jabber. "Can't you call my doctor and explain this to him? I can't follow anything you're saying. My brain is damaged."

I've started telling people I have a traumatic brain injury to increase the likelihood of understanding and compassion. What I tell them is technically true. A concussion is a mild traumatic brain injury. But the response I get from people when I say "brain injury" versus "concussion" is dramatic.

As expected, the woman agrees to call my primary care physician to explain the correct coding.

When the call ends, I put my phone aside and cry.

My husband strides into the room. "What's wrong?"

I tell him everything. He grabs his keys, wallet, and phone from the kitchen counter. "I'll go down and take care of it," he says. "I can't have you being this way forever."

Before the referral for neurological rehabilitation was made, my husband and I visited his oldest friend's wife who had recovered from a concussion five years ago. She told us where she went and what type of therapy she received. "You need to act now," she said. "The longer you wait, the less likely you will fully recover."

She told us the statistics. When a concussion lasts longer than three to six months, only twenty-seven percent of patients show noticeable improvement, leaving seventy-three percent of patients permanently disabled.

It's been five months.

When my husband returns an hour later, he hands me a piece of paper with my first appointment. My heart swells with hope and gratitude. I fling my arms around his neck and kiss him. "Thank you so much," I say.

Balancing Spoons

The physical therapist is more than an experienced concussion expert. She has personally recovered from a concussion twice.

Every week, we go through a set of exercises I practice twice a day at home. Every week, she tests my body's responses. "You're progressing well," she says.

My balance has improved. So has my depth perception. But my endurance is lagging. I nap every afternoon. When I overdo things, I wake up with symptoms all over again.

"You need to increase your spoons," she says.

"Spoons?"

She explains the concept of energy using teaspoons. Everyone has a limited number of teaspoons to use each day. Healthier people have more teaspoons. People recovering from injuries have less teaspoons. "A brain injury is different because no one can see how bad the injury is since you look normal. It's not like a broken arm, but it's worse than a broken arm. You can put a cast on an arm and force it to heal. You can't brace your brain and allow it the time it needs to heal. You are always using your brain even when you're doing nothing." She pauses, waiting for me to catch up with my understanding. "Everything we do either takes away or adds to our collection of spoons. For example, reading for fifteen minutes takes away one spoon, but enjoying a bubble bath gives one spoon. The key is to always have more spoons than you're spending. If you spend too many spoons, you'll wake up with symptoms."

The following weeks, I track my energy in spoons. Does this increase my energy? Or does it decrease my energy?

Even after I run out of therapy appointments (the insurance only approved five when I probably needed ten), I still struggle balancing spoons. Some days are better than others. But no day is perfect.

How many spoons do you have?

Too Much

As soon as I open my eyes, pain shoots through them.
I snap them shut, roll over in bed, and groan.
What did I do yesterday that pushed me over my limits?

Was it vacuuming and dusting the house?
Was it playing the home decorating game on my phone?
Was it grocery shopping after going to the gym?

Testing my body's abilities is a balancing act
Like juggling what I want to do against what I can
And never knowing when it is too much until tomorrow.

If I wake up without any symptoms,
I did well yesterday.
But if I hear ringing in my ears,
Feel shooting pain in my eyes, or
Breathe through congestion in my nose,
I did too much.

I have to toggle back, adjust my expectations, maybe
Cancel an appointment, lie down, rest, do nothing
Until I wake with no symptoms, and start again.

Attachment

The Buddhist believe all suffering comes from attachment. Attachment is clinging, and clinging is a klesha. To let go is to detach, which is to release suffering.

I am remembering these Buddhist teachings as I am contemplating which painting to give a friend who is recovering from cancer treatment, which is its own suffering.

My preference is one of my lesser paintings, something small, not a failure, but not my best or personal favorite. But after surveying my options, I keep returning to the only one that resonates, which is *Book Birds*. My friend is a reader, and she would appreciate the bookcase and the birds flying from the mind like stories into the wind.

Even my husband, the amateur art critic, believes it is one of my finest works. The resistance I feel reveals my attachment. I can't let go, can't part with this creation without a bit of resentment and hostility.

But if I give her anything less, I give her nothing of myself. And so, I must reorient my mind and loosen my attachment.

Each artwork is only with me for a limited time, and my time with *Book Birds* is up. It has graced my bookcase for months, and now it must spend some moments with my friend to remind her of how much she means to me, how glad I am to know she has survived.

Now, when I think of the artwork, which she received with

heartfelt gratitude, a surge of peace floods through me.

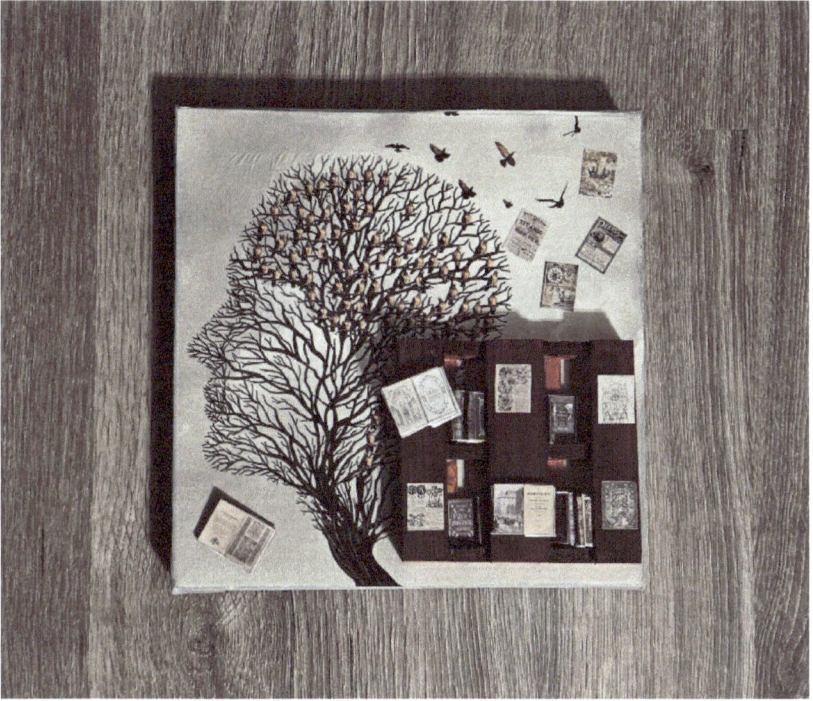

Book Birds, 8" X 8", mixed media

Talk Therapy 2

This week when I meet with Peter, I tell him about the group text I received from my stepdaughter over the weekend about her finishing the San Francisco Marathon.

I choke up when I tell him about my typed response:

—*I envy you. I don't know if I'll ever run again.*—

My comment was met with silence.

Moments later, I sent an apology.

—*Sorry. Not the same since concussion. Congrats on placing in the top ten for all women runners.*—

After I sent the text, I promptly deleted the group text chain.

Peter listens and nods. "You handled it well," he says. "You caught your mistake and corrected your course. So, why are you crying?"

I gulp. "I don't miss competing. But I do miss running."

Peter shrugs. "Maybe when you're all better, you'll run again."

No one can tell me if I'll get all better or if I'll run again. "I'm grieving. I need help processing this grief."

"Grieving is easy," he says.

"Easy?" I don't know how processing a loss can be called "easy." So, I ask, "What do you mean?"

"You state your loss as a fact, and you use a physical gesture to signal to your body that you're letting go." He demonstrates by snapping his fingers and saying, "I accept I can't run."

I snap my fingers. "I accept I can't run." I repeat the statement like a parrot, but inside heaviness sinks deep into me, filling up every crevice, making my arms and legs impossible to move.

He glances at the clock on his computer screen and says, "We have to wrap this up," even though two weeks ago we ended early because we didn't have anything to say to each other anymore.

"Can't we stay a little bit longer to make up for the last session?" I ask.

Shaking his head, he says, "I have another appointment."

I know from seeing him for the past two months that the grim line of his lips means he is lying. He does not have an appointment except maybe with Finnegan and Alaska's nature.

"But I don't feel better." My hands close to fists, and my lungs burn. I want a beer and a burger and an afternoon to forget. "I feel worse." That part of my brain that is still broken, that controls my moods, unhinges, and I cry, "I could drink myself to death."

"You won't drink yourself to death," he says, matter-of-factly.

"How can you be so sure?" I narrow my eyes. Aren't therapists supposed to keep watch over you during these moments of crises?

"Because you'll learn to accept how you feel." He snaps his fingers.

But as soon as the session ends, I drive to the gas station and buy a beer. I go next door to the 24-hour fast food joint and buy a burger. I've recently started eating solid food and drinking whatever I feel like, and my body has responded by gaining more weight than I previously lost. Two sips into the drink and two bites into the burger, my mind sparks and fizzles. Peter is right. I can't drink myself to death. That old buzz I wanted to feel, the one that makes my limbs floaty, and my tongue feel full, doesn't happen. I go straight from sober to hung over with a hammering headache that reminds me my brain is inflamed. My gut, used to fat-free soups and protein shakes, cramps from the greasy burger. I spend the rest of the afternoon in the bathroom.

When I finally emerge, I don't feel better. I feel much worse.

I dump the rest of the beer into the kitchen sink, shove the half-eaten burger into the trash, and send an email to the psychologist, telling him what I've done, and what I want to do. "I broke my sobriety. I never want to see you again."

Ten minutes later, he responds.

"Don't you want to have at least one more session?"

I want to type, "Just accept!" But I know he will not see the irony of that statement, so I agree to one more meeting in two weeks.

While I wait, I try and practice acceptance, but all I return to is the list of losses stacked up like overdue bills on a kitchen counter, demanding attention.

How can I accept losing the life I once led?

How can I accept no longer being the old me?

The art, which saved my life, can't rebuild it.

What can?

When I think back to the things that previously helped me process grief in a healthy way, I think back to three things—running, talking with my ex-husband, and attending therapy. But I can't tolerate a 5-mile jog, my ex-husband is out of reach, and my therapist isn't helping.

What else can I do?

Think, think, think.

But it hurts to think.

When my father was living with advanced Parkinson's, he spent most of his days in bed. "How do you tolerate it?" I asked.

"I pray," he said.

I've been praying and meditating every day for months. But I still haven't reached acceptance. Buddhists talk about impermanence, how everything is always changing. They believe all you take with you when you die is your state of mind, but I know that's not true from my experience of being disconnected from my mind while living. They say clinging causes suffering, but detaching causes relief.

Am I attached to running? Will detaching bring relief?

Morning Mantra

Every day I listen to Lisa Meta on the Inside Timer app. "Good morning," she says, before launching into her two-minute motivational speech.

Over the months, I've internalized a lot of her message:

1. You are the creator of your life.
2. Take a deep breath.
3. Your best self needs you to show up today.
4. Reach high to achieve your goals and push past any resistance.
5. You can do it. If you say you can, you can. If you say you can't, you can't.
6. No task is too hard.
7. Just start.
8. You are amazing.
9. You are powerful.
10. You've already accomplished so much. Don't stop.
11. Make choices, not excuses.
12. I believe in you. Do you believe in you?

Yes, I believe in me.

My Cousin's Wedding

June. Santa Nella, California,
Hotel Mission De Oro.
Heat blazing, almost 100 degrees.
Men in tuxes, women in tulle.

Fifty-eight years old and newly married,
My cousin Eddie greets me at the reception.
We stand before the speakers, music blaring,
But all I hear is his love for me.

Six months ago, at St. Rose's Church,
I cowered in the hallway near the bathrooms,
Cupping hands over ears, desperate to stop
The cacophony of violins and laughter.

Now I can tolerate the noise of celebration.
I can hug my cousins, one after another,
Catch up with them about life,
From new jobs to new homes to new loves.

From the three o'clock ceremony beneath a baking sky
To the five o'clock dinner in the air-conditioned hall,
I party—eating chicken piccata and drinking
Two glasses of champagne.

Who cares if my head swells? I want to live
Like everyone else, if only for this moment.
I am tired of hiding in a dark, soundless room,
Wishing, hoping, praying for a miracle.

But by seven o'clock, my body surrenders.
I tell Eddie I need to lie down and rest.

Before I go, my husband snaps a picture of me
Wedged between bride and groom.

In our hotel room overlooking the courtyard,
Before falling asleep, I call my mother and text
My sisters who could not attend.
In the morning, I write in my journal:

My cousin feared he would be single forever.
Now he's happily married.
I need to stop fearing I will never be 100% better.
I need to believe complete healing is possible.

Back To Work

My boss calls to ask if I am ready to return to online teaching. I don't feel ready, but I don't have any more sick time and my doctor thinks I should give it a try.

So, I do.

I teach a beginner's six-week course in creative writing. I log into the classroom each morning, post my questions and responses on the virtual blackboard, and correct 500-word assignments.

Just like I do everything, I separate my workload into fifteen-minute increments. I continue this process each week.

Halfway through the course, I ask my boss for her opinion on how I'm doing.

She examines my classroom before she responds. "It's okay if your feedback is taking a bit longer since it's detailed and thoughtful," she says. "It's worth the wait."

But once the class ends, I am not assigned another course to teach. The days stretch out listlessly before me, and for the first time I wonder if my teaching career is over.

I begin to look for other employment, but no one wants to hire someone who must take a break every fifteen minutes. "I should start smoking," I joke with my friend, Betty. "Then I can take as many breaks as I need." She laughs.

My physical therapist says I should be grateful. "I tell all my patients to not do too much the first year of recovery. Your body needs time to fully heal." She goes on to share stories about patients who returned to playing their sport too soon, thus ending their careers, while others waited a year or two, and were able to play for years on end. "Which camp do you want to be in?" she asks.

"The one who plays forever," I say.

"Then don't be in a hurry to go back to work. Let your body rest."

And so, I rest.

Interrupted Sleep

Six months ago, I could not stay asleep for more than three hours. Now, I wake three hours later, remembering something that I forgot during the day—deleting the amount of salt needed from a recipe, cleaning the oven, writing down a new fact for my resume (even though no one has called me for an interview). I take care of what I can and crawl back into bed and start to drift off again, only to remember something more. Afraid I will forget, I scramble from underneath the covers and pad down the hallway into my office and write it down. When I return to bed, I vow to sleep. I pray, and when the prayers fail to make me drowsy, I reach for my headphones and listen to a deep sleep meditation. When that fails, I lie awake, hands folded over my chest, with a silky silver sleeping mask over my eyes, just breathing. I only know I've fallen back to sleep when I jar awake three hours later from a dream about being in a restaurant sitting on stools that double as toilets, about walking down a flight of stairs with a guy who wanted to date me in high school, about moving out of a house while the next family moves in. I claw out of bed, wobbly and dizzy, needing more sleep, but unable to return to bed because the day has already begun, and I don't want to be late for my final meeting with the therapist.

Talk Therapy 3

Closure. This meeting is about closure.

Not for me, but for Peter.

When his face fills the screen, he leans back in the trailer with the sun blazing through the passenger's side window. I can see Finnegan loping in the distance between the stark trees, a glittering river in the distance.

"Thank you for agreeing to this final meeting," he says.

"Of course." I have former friends who worked as therapists, and from them I learned the importance of closure.

But my journey doesn't end after Peter gives me a list of things to do to stay sober (taking baths, long walks with husband, praying and meditating, art) and things to avoid (overworking, junk food, caffeine, not enough sleep). I am just starting to write about the moments before that fateful fall to the moments of this final meeting and beyond. Always beyond. Because the words will take me where I want to go if I trust them. For forty years, I've trusted the writing process. It has never failed me. It won't fail now.

Goodbye Old Me, Hello New Me

Saying goodbye to the person I was before the concussion was like giving up hope for a comeback story where the hero triumphs over adversity to regain a former glory. Like Rocky winning the boxing championship. Or the Karate Kid taking his opponent down.

Occasionally, a story from your life abruptly ends with no second chance for another victory. It's hard not to think of it as failure.

"I retired from running altogether in 2022," Beth Adair, a 58-year-old fitness guru, said in a statement for *Strong Fitness Magazine*. She has moved on to other things to stay fit and healthy like tracking her protein, eating clean, and staying consistent with her abdominal workouts. Always have a goal to train for, she advises.

She volunteers on occasion at running events to stay in touch with the running community even though she no longer runs.

But to do that I would have to be okay with not running, okay with being around others who are running, and focus on the positive energy of the race day without becoming overwhelmed in grief. I would have to say goodbye to the old me and hello to the new me.

Can I do it?

Not yet. But maybe someday I will.

In the article, Beth says her goals remain the same—getting stronger and staying stronger as the years progress—even though the means to the end have changed.

How can I find a way to achieve my goal—maintaining my weight and managing my moods—even though the avenue I once traveled to get there has closed (running and weight training)?

"I want to keep as much muscle as I can moving into my sixties," Beth said. "I can't imagine not working out."

But I know what not working out looks like while recovering from a concussion, and even though I can do more than a thirty-minute walk two times a day, I may never regain the mileage I lost. And that's okay, as long as I find another way to accomplish my goals.

Rejection

The first story I wrote after the concussion,
The one I shared with my husband
Who said it was about love and something else
Was rejected from the first publication I sent it to.

Normally, I would not feel a thing.
Okay, a twinge of sadness, maybe a hint of loss,
But since my brain doesn't work the same way,
The process was different this time.

This time I felt cracked open, exposed, a nerve
Twitching in the sunlight.

"That's normal," Nicole explained. "I feel gutted every time a piece is rejected. The more personal the piece, the more dejected I feel. Even though I know it's not personal."

"So, you're saying I'm normal?"

She laughs. "More normal than you've been in a long, long time."

Reading Again

"So, you're reading 400-to-600-page books?" my brother-in-law asks when he visits ten months after the concussion.

My eyes widen. "No, more like 200-to-300-page books, fifteen minutes at a time, for two to three hours a day, for a finish time of two to three weeks."

He nods, acknowledging the difference. "But it must be good to be reading again."

"It is," I say. Nine months ago, in the thick of my soupy brain, I mourned the loss of reading. Now I am savoring books I never thought I would enjoy, mostly classics I didn't have to read in high school, like *Lolita* and *The Color Purple*, as well as some recently published books to help my students who are preparing to query, and a couple on the bestseller list like *The Housemaid*. I must be careful not to overdo it, which is hard, especially if the writing is good. "One more chapter," I say to myself, even though my eyes are tiring.

"You should read *Elevation* by Stephen King," my brother-in-law says. "It's short. Your husband read it in one sitting."

The volume is 146 pages, which is nothing for a Stephen King book, which can be over a thousand pages like *The Stand*. But I'm not a huge fan of Stephen King, and the reading feels like a chore.

"You'll like it," my brother-in-law promises.

So, I accept the gift of borrowing his copy. That night I step inside a world where a man is mysteriously losing weight although externally, he appears as if nothing has changed. My scalp prickles. I identify with the main character. We both have something wrong with us that no one can see. We both need a solution to a problem that appears to have no answers.

My fingers turn the page, and my mind focuses.

My brother-in-law is right.

I like this story.

I like this character.

I am so thankful I can read again.

Art Therapy 3

I sell "Evening at the Opera" at the Santa Rosa Art Center during the Black and White Exhibit.

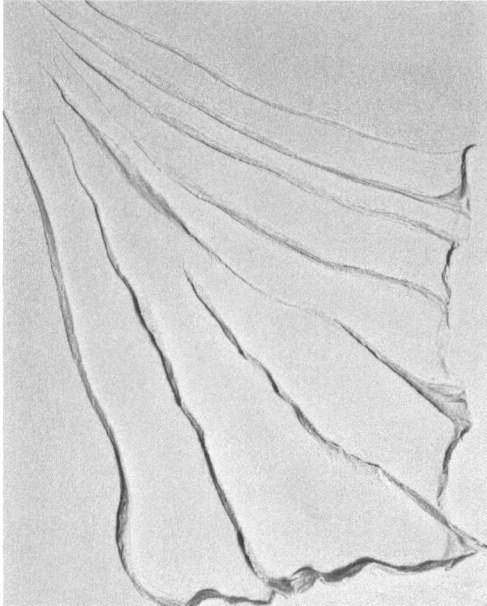

Evening at the Opera, 14" X 11", mixed media

Afterward, my husband asks what my cut is.

"Sixty-forty," I say.

"Could you do better if you sold elsewhere?" he asks.

I decide to look online to see if anyone is taking artists on consignment. I search a local gift shop that has been voted the best in Sonoma County several years in a row and fill out an application with links to my artwork posted online. I figure it will be like selling at Best Wishes only better.

A few weeks later, as my husband and I are driving to Carmel for a much-needed getaway, I receive an email congratulating me on my acceptance as the newest maker at Made Local.

When I return from our trip, I bring the originals I had posted online to the shop's owner. She shows me where she will display my artwork, on the back wall with several other local artists. "We need different price points," she explains. "Most of our sales are under $100." She shows me examples from my competitors: gift cards, magnets, and prints. I cringe. I had only wanted to sell my originals. I didn't want to start a whole line of artwork again. Twenty years ago, I sold on consignment at Best Wishes, a gift store, until the business closed. "If you bring in other items, I'll let you bring your books, even though books never sell," she says.

I do have tons of books stacked in a closet. My husband says I have to get rid of most of my collection before we move to our forever home, which will close escrow soon.

After deciding to go ahead with the consignment offer, I ask my fellow cohorts of the online art classes I've been taking if they know of a reputable place where I can get prints made. Over the course of a couple of weeks, I learn how to take professional quality photos of my artwork and convert the files into high resolution prints. I send one to Leanne, my former sister-in-law (who I consider a sibling). The canvas print is a replica of an acrylic painting from my trip to Puerto Rico.

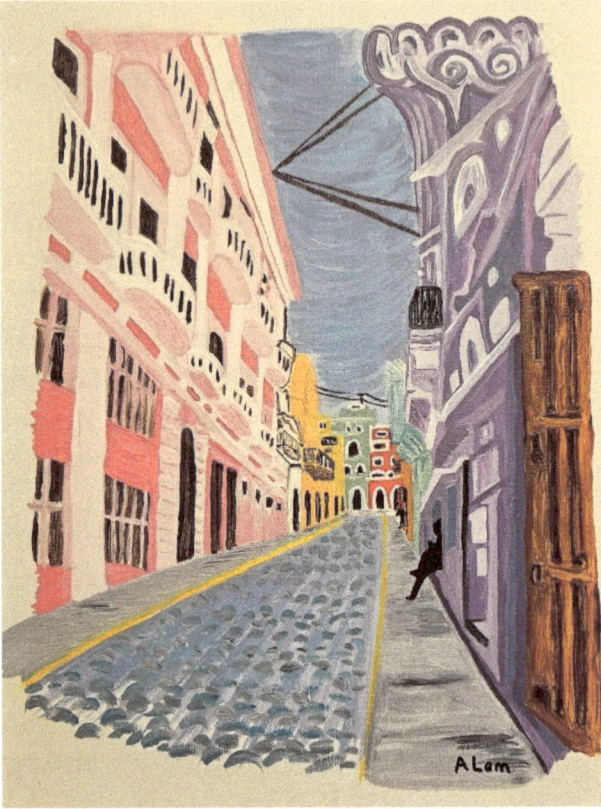

Puerto Rico, 14" X 11", acrylic on canvas

I find the painting of a swamp, which my youngest sister, Sylvia, said she wanted years ago. When I originally painted it on canvas paper, I didn't know how to copy and ship it to her. Now I do. I send her the same size canvas print as an early birthday present. When it arrives, she texts to let me know she can hardly wait to hang it in her home.

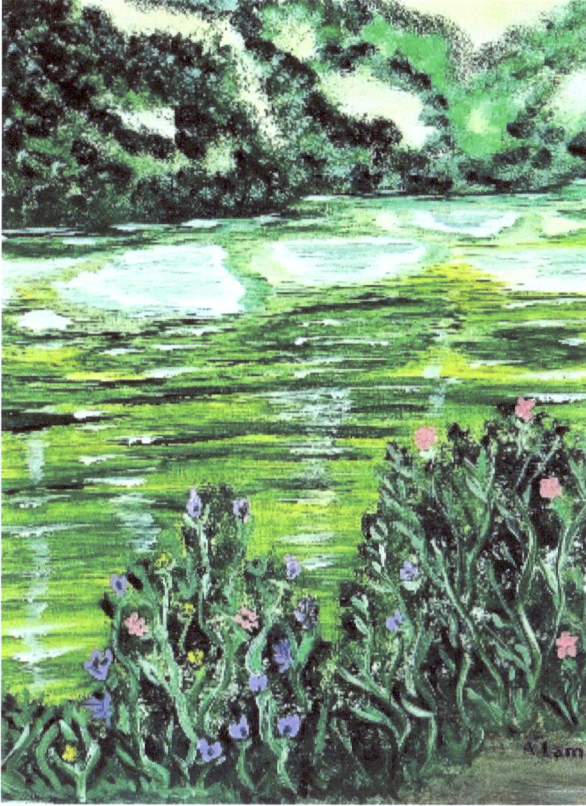

Swamp, 18" X 24", acrylic on paper canvas

I order materials to make smaller artworks in the $5 to $10 price range. The work is tedious. My husband and my daughter help with sticking price tags on sale items. I make greeting cards and magnets between time spent caring for my son and time spent lying on the sofa doing nothing.

Nothing sells the first month.

During the second month, I attend a "Meet and Greet the Maker" event but only stay for a couple of hours. Tucked away at the back of the store, I don't meet or greet many customers, but I do avoid the fanfare of live music and noisy chatter, which would only drain me.

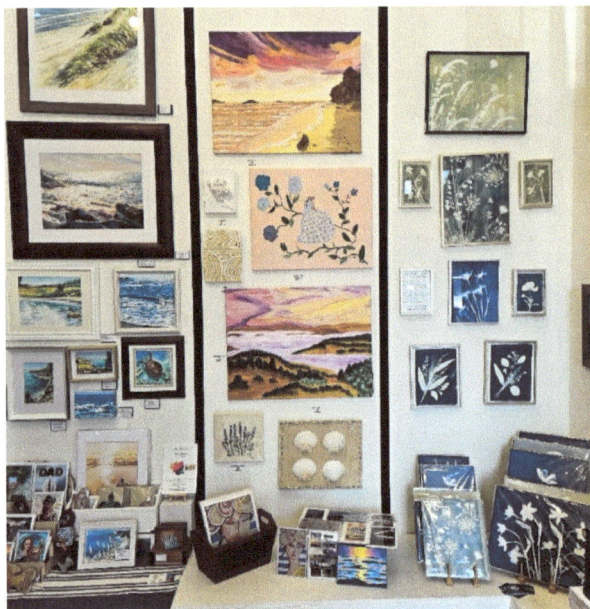

My Art Wall (center) at Made Local

Then, at the end of that second month, I stop by the store and notice one of my paintings is no longer on the wall. My heartbeat leaps in my chest. Finally, a sale! That piece of artwork, which I thought of as a homage to a woman who had undergone breast cancer and survived, was called, "Diva #4" of my four-piece Diva collection. Excited, I can hardly wait for the end-of-the-month email tallying the store's sales. When the anticipated email arrives, it states I have sold nothing. Nothing? I go to the store and talk to the owner. We examine the wall, confirm the painting is missing, and come to the only logical conclusion—it was shoplifted.

"Do you have business liability insurance?" the owner asks.

"You can file a claim."

Even if I did, the painting isn't worth the deductible.

I feel gutted, once again, just like I felt the first time my artwork was stolen after a district-wide art contest I won when I was in middle school.

That event created a setback so great, I didn't pick up a paintbrush for twenty years.

This time, I take the loss in stride. I vent to my husband and post a rant online.

I refuse to quit. I don't want to go back into the art closet, creating for an audience of one. I want to share my artwork with the world, so I soldier on.

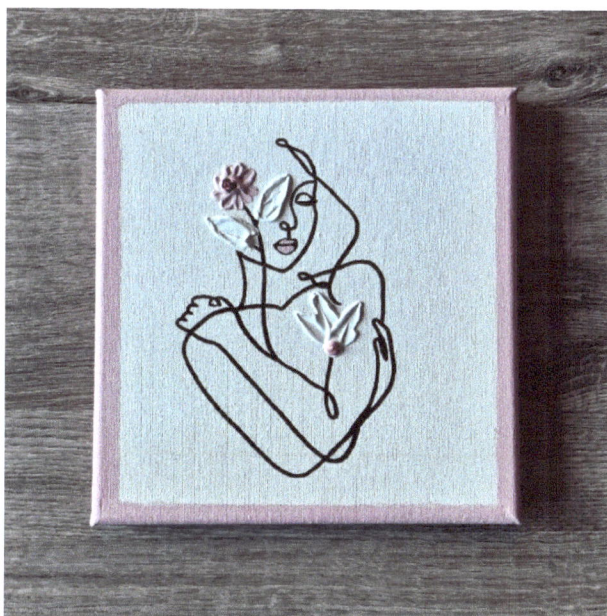

Diva #4, 8" X 8," mixed media

Sales start to happen shortly after my online rant. I look into getting business liability insurance. By the third month, I am making sales. I stock the store with bigger paintings and a handful of smaller originals that I know will probably get stolen. Loss leaders, I think, just like big retailers have. I even sell a couple of copies of my chapbook, *Water Baby and Other Stories*. I designed the book cover, too.

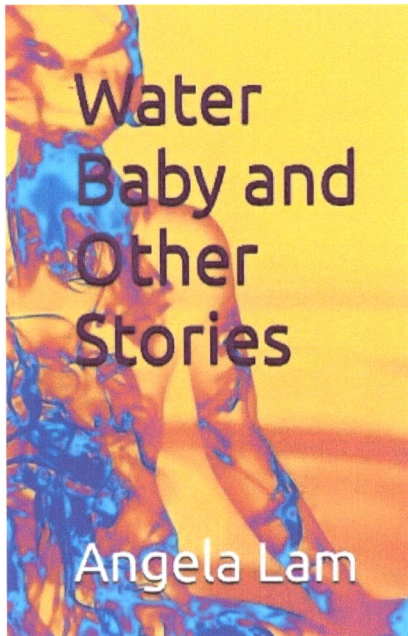

Despite a great third month of sales, by the fourth month, I receive the dreaded email from the owner. I have failed to sell the minimum needed to justify leasing the space to me.

I'm asked to leave.

I pack up my inventory and gift a small piece of work to the employee who helps me.

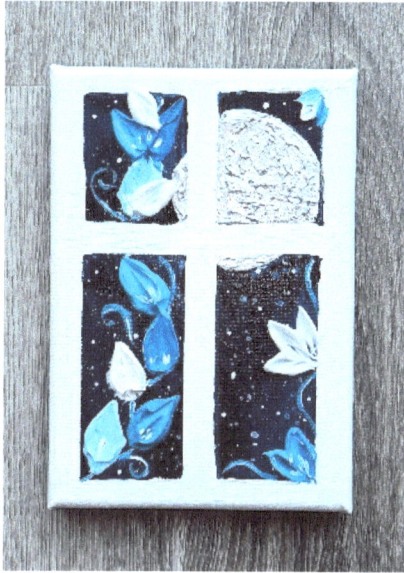

Goodnight Moon, 5" X 7", mixed media

I end this chapter of my artist life, much the way I ended it the first time around, with the quiet chime of the retail store door closing behind me.

At lunch with Betty, I tell her about the experience.

"Maybe you could teach art," she suggests. "I go to those Sip and Paint events once a month. It doesn't require much talent."

"They're franchises," I tell her. "I don't have twenty thousand sitting around, do you?"

"Not since my divorce," she says. "But maybe you could ask one of those people who own a franchise if you could work for them."

"Maybe," I agree. But I don't imagine I would earn a living subbing as a painting instructor.

When the Luther Burbank Center for the Arts offers a teaching certification course that would allow me to teach art anywhere in Sonoma County, I look into the program, which is designed for working artists seeking another avenue of income, which describes my situation perfectly. Additionally, the program is designed for busy professionals, requiring I only attend an in-person class two hours a week over a period of three months followed by a paid practicum.

After the lunch with Betty, I apply for the program. Within a week, I receive an acceptance.

A new chapter in my artistic journey has begun.

Return Of The Fair-Weather Friend

While I am painting a blue gray ombre on a canvas, my phone rings in the other room. With paint on my hands, I swipe the screen with the back of a knuckle. "Hello?"

Emma chirps. "I haven't talked to you in a while. I feel like we're falling out of touch."

I press the speaker button with the same knuckle, then turn the water on to rinse my hands in the sink. "It's good to hear from you," I say. I don't want to tell her I had written her off.

"I got your emails. What's this about a move?" she asks.

Three months ago, I sent her an email about my life— writing an offer on a house in Windsor, teaching my first class since the concussion, inviting her to attend an author reading and book signing with me. I share the story of our new home, and from there the conversation meanders until we end up talking about envy. "I'm envious of you," Emma says. "You have talent and the ability to get the writing done."

Her comment isn't new, but how I feel is. "I can't write the way I used to. I'm thankful I can read again. But when I read, I no longer think, 'I wish I could write like that.' Instead, I think, 'I'll never be able to write like that.' It's different. I don't have the ability, which feels worse than not having the talent. Does that make sense?"

"Oh, yes, but you're entitled to feel that way," Emma says. "My dad is almost 100. People say, 'You're doing so well,' but all he can think about is how much better he was just five years ago. He's lost his short-term memory, and he's no longer able to care for himself. He's lost what he once had, and that is why he's envious of others just like you're envious of other writers." She laughs. "I have no excuse for being envious of you. Except for needing more time." She must go.

After the call ends, a radiant warmth fills my chest. I'm not being unrealistic or pessimistic or a Debby Downer. I'm just feeling what anyone would feel in my situation. And Emma understands. I'm so thankful she called.

I've always told my writing students, "There will always be someone better than you and worse than you. Strive not to be better or worse than others but to have your writing be good enough for you." The same advice can apply to life, and it took Emma's call to remind me of that.

Setback

Nine months after the initial impact, my brain stutters and tangles up again. My scalp hurts. The left side of my face is congested. I can barely walk a straight line.

What's happening?

I think back to yesterday. What did I do differently? I scan my daily journal, but I find no clues. I don't write about every moment like I did in the beginning.

I play back the tape in my mind. Sleep? No, I had more than the previous night. Physical exertion? No, I had my son. We don't walk more than a few yards a handful of times a day, clearly less than the mile or so I walk with my husband. Food? I didn't eat too much or too little. So, what was it?

My daughter called. Twice. Once in the morning to announce she was divorcing. Once in the evening to say her husband had moved out and taken one of the three dogs, leaving the other two home alone for more than twelve hours. She was stuck at work, couldn't go to retrieve them, and I was stuck at home with my son, and I couldn't go to retrieve them either. What would they do? I never found out. She had to hang up and take a call from her husband.

That must be it. Emotional overload.

Before, I could tackle these types of situations. Yes, I might feel distress for my daughter, but I would not be paralyzed by neurological overwhelm. Now an emotionally charged event ricochets through my body sending seismic disturbances from my head to my feet. I lie down on the sofa. I close my eyes. I try to sleep. But nothing helps.

So, I take another approach. I text my daughter and ask about what happened.

She responds. Yes, her husband came home. Yes, he took care of the dogs. Yes, she would talk to him and sort things out regarding the future, whether they would go their separate ways, attend counseling, or just carry on.

Satisfied, I take a nap and wake up feeling not much better. But as the afternoon elongates into evening, I find my stride again. It is just like the beginning where my mornings were more difficult than the afternoons.

Only one thought continues to haunt me.

Will I always be this fragile? Or will I find my strength again?

Getting Better

Nicole and I hike up the paved path toward Spring Lake. We talk about the things we love— reading and writing. It is how we process life, make sense of the chaos, heal the brokenness, recover.

I tell her about the failed talk therapy, and she tells me about her trip to Prince Edward Island. I tell her about my experience terminating a publishing agreement, and she tells me about revising her 80,000-word manuscript before the September deadline.

Our legs move without assistance, and our breathing evens. I notice my diminished lung capacity from my inability to run, but Nicole only comments on my endurance. "You walked farther than you did last time!" I hear the pride and astonishment in her voice.

When our time together ends, we hug goodbye. She's headed to Sundance, and I'm headed nowhere. None of that matters. Our friendship is tethered to something greater than travel or stasis. It is rooted in love.

Relax

"I wasn't sure if I should have canceled my appointment since I'm still recovering from a concussion, and I don't see the same way anymore," I say, sitting in the exam chair in the eye clinic.

My doctor glances at the computer screen to read my file, then he faces me. "I had a concussion," he says. "It took a year and a half to recover. Looks like you're at the end of nine months. Is it any better?"

My whole-body tingles. This guy understands. He's had a concussion. He's recovered. I'm suddenly thankful I didn't cancel my appointment. I shift in the chair, so I am sitting taller. "I feel like I've plateaued. I still wake with pain in my left eye, and I still need an afternoon nap. My body tires so I break everything into fifteen-minute increments. I can't do anything for longer than three hours including teaching. I tried over the summer, and I wasn't asked back."

He examines my file again. "Everybody's different," he says. "I had blurry vision for the longest time. I tried everything, but nothing worked except meditation. I meditate in the morning, noon, and night. Do you meditate?"

I remember those days in the early months when all I could do was meditate. "Not so much anymore."

"You need to relax so your brain can heal because it is always working."

Relax. That word sticks with me. That's why making art has been crucial. It is my way of relaxing.

He asks how I got the concussion, and I ask how he got his. "I was hit by a car while biking. My helmet cracked. I was unconscious."

"Oh, my," I gasp. That's how the singer, Amy Grant, got her concussion—while biking. She hit a pothole and tumbled over the handlebars and cracked her helmet. She was also unconscious. She still struggles with her memory and must use a teleprompter when she performs so she knows the lyrics she sings even though she wrote them years ago. "Do you bike anymore?"

"Oh, yes, and I've started running. I couldn't do it at first because it was too jarring, but now I run more than I bike. I run on the surface streets too, but I am careful to stop before I get tired. I tend to drag my feet when I'm fatigued, so I don't want to trip and fall. The medical research shows you're more vulnerable to another concussion after you have one. But you need to exercise. Exercise helps everything."

I nod, knowing the statistics. The vestibular issues don't get better with age only worse. And I agree—exercise helps. I tell him about my twice daily walks with my husband. He suggests trying to run or bike to increase my endurance.

"You might also want to try those drug store readers at the lowest magnification. Even though you don't need reading glasses, they might help build your stamina."

It is worth a try, so I tell him I will try.

"You're doing the right thing by not working till you're completely healed," he says. "I wish I had taken more time off. I think I would have healed quicker."

I leave the appointment with renewed hope of speeding up my recovery through taking his advice.

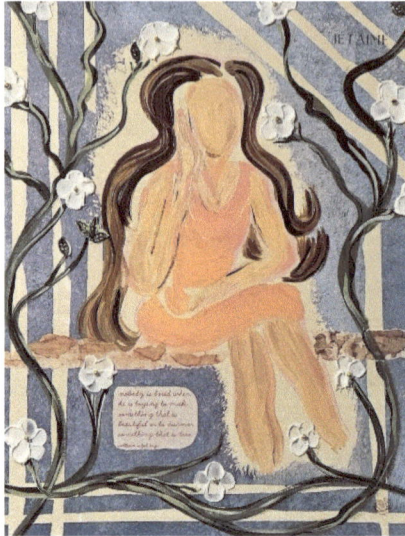

Beautiful and True, 30" X 24", mixed media

Return Of Monkey Mind

The Buddhists call the chattering thoughts that drift through your mind during a sitting meditation "monkey mind."

For the longest time, I could not think. Every time I tried, a tightness stretched across my forehead, wrapped itself around my skull, and squeezed. Sometimes it knocked or thudded. But it always, always resurrected in some form of pain. So, I learned not to think.

Now, as I am healing, I have noticed a return of monkey mind.

It starts out with a smattering of chatter like distant birds chirping, then evolves into distinct words that rush through my mind. *Do this, do that, how about this, how about that. Blah-blah-blah-blah-blah-blah-blah.*

Sometimes I can silence it. But the healthier I get, the harder it is to quiet those voices. A chorus of demands rings out, loud and clear, and I fall under its spell, obey its orders, lose myself in its senseless chatter. I become what I once was—a flawed human trying to quiet my mind—instead of who I thought I had become—a broken individual coasting on the waves of universal consciousness while waiting to be made whole again through the medical community. I am monkey mind again, and monkey mind is me.

Confession

Ten months after my concussion, I see my primary care physician for my annual wellness exam.

"How are you doing?" he asks.

"I'm fine," I say. The barometric pressure has changed with the autumn rain, which increases my headaches, but not enough to keep me home. "I drove thirty minutes in morning traffic to make the appointment."

"That's great," he says. "The last time I saw you, your husband had driven you."

That's right. He did.

"You know, for a while I doubted you would get better," he confesses. "It was taking so long to see any sign of improvement."

Thankfully, there has been lots of improvement since that initial appointment.

1. I can read.
2. I can write for 30 minutes at a time.
3. I can watch a movie in a theater.
4. I can dine in a noisy restaurant.
5. I can exercise.
6. I can clean the house.
7. I can sleep.
8. I can work part-time.

Sure, I sometimes need an afternoon nap, and sometimes I wake with stabbing pain in my left eye or with a loss of balance so great I feel like I'm drunk although I am sober. But for the most part, I am better—better than my primary care physician thought I would be.

And, for once in my life, better is good enough for me.

Better Broken*

Almost a year after the concussion, I sit on the bench in the foyer putting on my shoes to go for a walk with my husband. My thoughts circle back to a playful conversation we had last night with his brother about how defective I am and is it too late to get a refund on the new wife warranty. I know it was friendly banter (my brother-in-law is a professional comedian), but that insecure part of me still asks my husband, "Do you wish I had stayed forty or do you just wish I was healthy again?"

My husband's eyes glaze over. "Both," he mumbles.

"What?" I repeat.

"Just get better," he snaps.

Eight months ago, I lay on the sofa wondering if I would be useless for the rest of my life.

My thirty-year-old mute son glanced up from the floor where he was sitting, tearing up pages from a catalogue, and tucked a piece of paper into my hand.

I stared at the photo of a pendant inscribed with the words, "Never, never, never give up." The endless days battling doctors who didn't understand and insurance that wouldn't pay floated away, and a bright glow of determination filled my chest. "Okay." I smiled and kissed his cheek. "I will."

That feeling returns to my body even as a headache ripples beneath my scalp. "I'll get better," I tell my husband, not a promise, but a reassurance. "I'll run again, lose the weight, be the old me again."

My husband shakes his head, as if he knows the future. "You'll never be the same."

I think back to the art class I took at the beginning of the year, how the instructor told us it was okay to not be perfect. "Wabi-sabi," she said, pointing to a squiggly, unmanageable line that made the work look better. "You want things natural. That's what differentiates us from AI. Our imperfections are what makes us unique and our artwork valuable."

Outside, in the crisp morning air, I take my husband's hand, and we stroll through our new neighborhood. I want to remind him about the sculpture we saw in Carmel in the spring, how it had broken into many pieces. Instead of throwing everything away and starting new, the artist installed a light inside the hollow core and glued together the pieces, leaving a few spots missing so the light could shine through. That's how I imagine my healing to be, perfectly imperfect, a work of art, made more beautiful by brokenness. But I say nothing, just squeeze his hand, and walk a little faster to keep the pace.

*A portion of this piece appeared in *Five Minutes*